YOUR KNOWLEDGE HAS VALUE

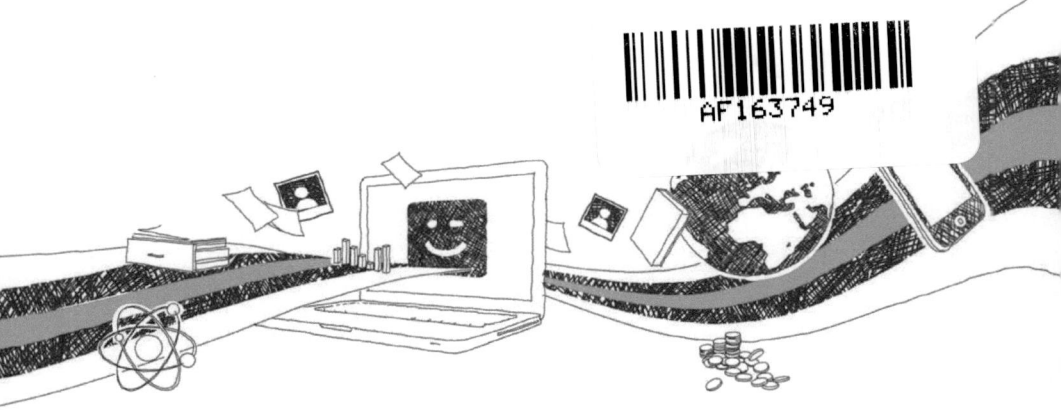

- We will publish your bachelor's and master's thesis, essays and papers

- Your own eBook and book - sold worldwide in all relevant shops

- Earn money with each sale

Upload your text at www.GRIN.com
and publish for free

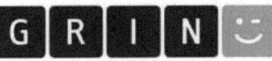

Alikira Richard

Adoption of clinical information systems in hospitals in Uganda

GRIN Publishing

Bibliographic information published by the German National Library:

The German National Library lists this publication in the National Bibliography; detailed bibliographic data are available on the Internet at http://dnb.dnb.de .

This book is copyright material and must not be copied, reproduced, transferred, distributed, leased, licensed or publicly performed or used in any way except as specifically permitted in writing by the publishers, as allowed under the terms and conditions under which it was purchased or as strictly permitted by applicable copyright law. Any unauthorized distribution or use of this text may be a direct infringement of the author s and publisher s rights and those responsible may be liable in law accordingly.

Imprint:

Copyright © 2012 GRIN Verlag GmbH
Print and binding: Books on Demand GmbH, Norderstedt Germany
ISBN: 978-3-656-35728-5

This book at GRIN:

http://www.grin.com/en/e-book/208148/adoption-of-clinical-information-systems-in-hospitals-in-uganda

GRIN - Your knowledge has value

Since its foundation in 1998, GRIN has specialized in publishing academic texts by students, college teachers and other academics as e-book and printed book. The website www.grin.com is an ideal platform for presenting term papers, final papers, scientific essays, dissertations and specialist books.

Visit us on the internet:

http://www.grin.com/

http://www.facebook.com/grincom

http://www.twitter.com/grin_com

Adoption of clinical information systems in hospitals in Uganda

A proposal submitted to the school of postgraduates Studies and research in partial fulfillment for the Award of the degree of doctor of Management of information Systems

BY

Richard, A

April, 2012

CONTENTS

- CONTENTS 2
- LIST OF FIGURES AND TABLES 3
- EXECUTIVE SUMMARY 4
- CHAPTER ONE 5
- THE PROBLEM AND ITS SCOPE 5
  - 1.1 Background of the study 5
  - 1.2 Statement of the problem 9
  - 1.3 Purpose of the study 9
  - 1.4 Research objectives 10
  - 1.5 Research questions 10
  - 1.6 Hypothesis 10
  - 1.7 Scope of the Study 10
  - 1.8 Significance of the study 11
  - 1.9 Operational definitions 12
- CHAPTER TWO 13
- LITERATURE REVIEW 13
  - 2.1 Requirements analysis 13
  - 2.2 System design techniques 15
  - 2.3 The Role of Physicians and Barriers to Use 16
  - 2.4 Benefits of the Clinical Information Systems 16
- CHAPTER THREE 20
- METHODOLOGY 20
  - 3.1 Research Design 20
  - 3.2 Study population 21
  - 3.3 Target Sample 24
    - 3.3.1 Sampling procedure 24
  - 3.4 Data collection tools 24
  - 3.5 Scoring of the scale 25
  - 3.6 Validity and reliability of the instrument 25
  - 3.7 Data Gathering Procedures 26
  - 3.8 Data Analysis 27
  - 3.8 Ethical Considerations 27
  - 3.9 Limitations of the study 28
  - References 29

APPENDIX II 32
   QUESTIONAIRE... 32

LIST OF FIGURES AND TABLES

Figure 3.1: showing the distribution of hospitals in Uganda..21
Figure 3.2: showing Yamane's formula for calculating target.......................................24
Table 3.1: The table below shows Health workers at national level..............................22
Table 3.2: Table showing the estimated total population stratified..............................23

EXECUTIVE SUMMARY

Clinical information systems offer the possibility to improve healthcare quality by providing clinical task support and clinical decision support by influencing clinical decisions at the time and place that these decisions are made. Unfortunately hospitals in Uganda have for long neglected their use despite mounting pressure from medical workers seeking pay rise which has left most government hospitals understaffed. As a result, patients are not attended to on time and medical trainees who assist in most hospitals sometimes lack the desired skills and do not get adequate guidance from experienced health workers to enable them make more informed decisions. The purpose of this study is to evaluate the use of CIS in improving the quality of health care by providing clinical task support to medical workers. Data will be collected from mainly health workers working regional referral hospitals in Uganda whose populace is estimated to be 9000 and 383 will be sampled and given questionnaires. Depending on the outcome from the study, recommendations will be made on whether the government of Uganda should adopt clinical information systems in Uganda.

CHAPTER ONE
THE PROBLEM AND ITS SCOPE

1.1 Background of the study

The health care market is the largest industry in the United States, with expenditures of about $2.6 trillion, or 15.9% of the national GDP in 2010. The rapid increase in health care expenditures, technology has developed to provide support to health care delivery staff. The primary care delivery entity is the physician or the specialist. Throughout the evolution of medical technology, the development of an efficient, useful, and practical clinical information system has become a significant focus in the vendor market. However, the resistance to the implementation of helpful technology that is common within the health care market has limited the maximization of the potential of clinical information systems. Through the satisfaction of aggregate physician needs in conjunction with the needs of health care managers, the implementation of a clinical information system can be advantageous to the health care delivery process.

The school dictionary defines a decision as settlement or conclusion reached based on certain data. According to George, Robert, Brent & Eugene (2001), DSSs are used in the identification of problems or decision making opportunities (similar to exception reporting), identification of possible solutions or decisions, provision of access to information needed to solve a problem or make a decision, analysis of possible decisions or of variances that will affect a decision. Sometimes this is called "what if....." analysis, and Simulation of possible solutions. Shortliffe, Scott, Bischoff, Campbell &Melle (1981), a CDSS refers to any computer programme that helps health professionals to make clinical decisions. Their definition has a disadvantage that it includes any computer system presenting medical knowledge, including the World Wide Web or electronic textbooks. A better definition should take into account the application to patient care and the intent of the CDSS to give case-specific advice. Thus, A clinical information system is a collection of various information technology applications that provides a centralized repository of information related to patient care across distributed locations. This repository represents the patient's history of illnesses and interactions with providers by encoding knowledge capable of helping clinicians decide about the patient's condition, treatment options, and wellness activities. The repository also encodes the status of decisions, actions underway for those decisions, and relevant information that can help in performing those actions. The database could also hold other information about the patient, including genetic, environmental, and social contexts.

According to Gluud & Nikolova (2007), in the early 1970s the first computerized general practice system was produced in the United States, which resulted in a standard computer-generated prescription form. By 1989, a proportion of general practice information technology (IT) investment became directly remunerable and computer use became widespread.

Kawamoto, Caitlin, Houlihan, Andrew, David & Lobach (2005), define a CDSS as, an application that analyzes data to help healthcare providers make clinical decisions. It is an adaptation of the decision support system commonly used to support business management. Physicians, nurses and other health care professionals use a CDSS to prepare a diagnosis and to review the diagnosis as a means of improving the final result. Data mining may be conducted to examine the patient's medical history in conjunction with relevant clinical research. Such analysis can help predict potential events, which can range from drug interactions to disease symptoms. They provide clinicians, staff, patients, and other individuals with knowledge and patient specific information, intelligently filtered and presented at appropriate times, to enhance health services. Since 2004, when the Federal Government promoted the importance of electronic medical records there has been a slow but increasing adoption of HIT, to improve the quality of health services. World over, and specifically in the US, Europe, Asia and to a small extent in Africa, HIT is being regarded the cheapest way of boosting human resource especially in the health industry. Germany was the first country to start developing a national HIT network in 1993. In 1997, Canada established the Advisory Council on Health Infrastructure and in 2001 launched Canada Health Infoway, a nonprofit organization. By the end of 2009, Canada Health Infoway had half its population using the EHRs.

In south Africa and Libya, CDSS are a point-of-order decision aids, usually through computer order entry systems, that provide real-time feedback to health on which medical workers base to make diagnosis or even to give treatment to patients. In the journal of the American medical association (JAMA), it was published that most hospitals faced pressure cuts in government payments and demand for lower hospital fees and shorter hospital stays. Many have responded by reducing staff or employing few staff and merging with other institutions. Some teaching hospitals especially in the United States have taken these steps, but their problems are compounded by the extra obligations that they have long assumed such as training new physicians and other health care personnel, conducting medical research, and providing free care for the poor. Teaching hospitals shape the future of medicine by providing most of the clinical research in new procedures, technology, treatments, and medications and thus to fully achieve their obligations, there is need to provide enough assistance to both medical trainees and patients. And due to cost pressure, this has seen the introduction of systems like the internist which guide and may act as a virtual trainer to inexperienced medics.

Uganda is a landlocked country located in East Africa, just north of Lake Victoria, astride the equator. The country has a total area of 241,038 square kilometers of which 43 942 square kilometers are swamps and 197 096 square kilometres is land. The figures of 2002 Population and Housing Census indicate that Uganda's population grew at an average rate of 3.4% per annum between 1991 and 2002. From the National Census Report, Uganda has a projected population of 27.7 million people, and fertility rate of 6.9%. Infant Mortality Rate (IMR) stands at 88 per 1,000 live births while Maternal
Mortality Rate (MMR) is 506 per 100 000 births. The country is divided into 80 districts which are decentralized. Broadly these districts are divided into rural and urban

districts.

According to Joseph, Cissy, Mbasaalaki-Mwaka & Grace (2010), in their study on challenges faced by health workers in providing counseling services to HIV-positive children in Uganda, it was discovered that some of the challenges faced by hospitals include; limited staff leading to heavy workloads; shortage of testing kits and other logistics; lack of, or inadequate protection against occupational hazards like pricking and infections like tuberculosis; lack of comprehensive HIV/AIDS counseling; and lack of sensitization at health facilities prior sending patients to laboratories. For example; Mulago hospital which is a national hospital suffers from lack of enough personnel and so clients often queue for hours. Literary meaning if patients who really need immediate attention and cannot help themselves queue for hours, there is a high possibility of students not getting attention at all. They also found out that, a quarter of the health workers (14 of 59; 24%) were constrained by inadequate knowledge about pediatric HIV care and the lack of pediatric counseling skills. One health worker said "Some of us have never trained or even been trained in counseling." Many times, it happens that the people we expect to know do not know. This shows that students in teaching hospitals are not only faced by lack of teachers/instructors but they also lack instructors with adequate knowledge and experience.

According to the former minister of Health, Mike (2010), KIU teaching hospital has the highest number of patient beds in Uganda with 1,200; while Mulago Hospital, a national referral hospital has 1,000 and Butabika has 906. Despite the big number of beds at KIU-TH, it was discovered in a pilot study carried out in October of 2011 that the lecturer to student ratio had grown to 1:23 in the departments of health sciences contrary to the world wide accepted ratio of 1:8. Many other hospitals including Mulago that was built to support 906 patients currently support more than 10,000 patients. It is on this ground that a study should be undertaken to evaluate the effects of CIS on the performance of health workers and thereafter draw recommendations on whether CISs should be adopted in Ugandan hospitals.

1.2 Statement of the problem

Clinical information systems offer the possibility to improve healthcare quality by providing clinical task support and clinical decision support by influencing clinical decisions at the time and place that these decisions are made. Unfortunately hospitals in Uganda have for long neglected their use despite mounting pressure from medical workers seeking pay rise which has left most government hospitals understaffed. As a result, patients are not attended to on time and medical trainees who assist in most hospitals sometimes lack the desired skills and do not get adequate guidance from experienced health workers to enable them make more informed decisions. Lack of enough practical skills manifests itself when they fail to correlate signs and symptoms with diseases that cause them. Inadequate staff at Mulago hospital and other hospitals both government and private has significantly contributed to the poor services in hospitals. At KIU, students went on strike over the same issue of inadequate staff to guide them (Wilber, 2010) , at Amana hospital, a child died as the parents waited in the line for treatment (Richard,2006), similar cases are happening in many other small and big hospitals in Uganda and beyond unnoticed. It is common to find hospitals using more of trainees (who in most cases have partial ideas on treatment) than experienced health workers which puts patients' lives at risk. As a remedy, patients and students alike prefer consulting with experienced doctors who in most cases are not readily available. The time lag created delays patients, students and medical practitioners creating inefficiency in all hospital operations and on several occasions has resulted in loss of lives (Richard, thur Apr 13, 2006) in the IPP newspaper. It is because of the above that clinical information systems should be adopted to supplement the services of medical experts by providing medical trainees with fast access to knowledge acquired from various medical experts at the time and place of diagnosis so as to improve the quality of health care.

1.3 Purpose of the study

The purpose of this study is to evaluate the use of CIS in improving the quality of health care by providing clinical task support to medical workers.

1.4 Research objectives

1. To develop software requirements specification for a clinical information systems,
2. To investigate techniques used in designing clinical information system,
3. To assess the role of health workers in the implementation of clinical information systems,
4. And to evaluate the effects of clinical information systems on the efficiency of medical workers.

1.5 Research questions

What are software requirements for a clinical help system?

Which techniques can be used to design a clinical information system?

What role do health workers play in the implementation of clinical information systems?

What are the effects of using clinical information system on the efficiency medical workers?

1.6 Hypothesis

The use of clinical information systems improves the performance of inexperienced medical workers.

1.7 Scope of the Study

Geographically, the study will be carried out in Uganda specifically in the districts of; Arua, fort portal, Gulu, Hoima ,Jinja ,Kabale,Lira ,Masaka ,Mbale ,Soroti and Mubende . The above districts were selected because it is in them that regional referral hospitals are located.

The study will include; collection of data, development of software requirements specification for an appropriate clinical information system, evaluation of system design techniques, and assessment of the impact of using clinical information systems on the efficiency of medical workers.

Data will collected from medical workers from twelve regional referral hospitals. These hospitals serve hundreds of patients. People who interact with people having various health problems are the main target. They will include; Medical Doctors, clinicians nurses, medical students and administrative staff. Books, journals and online material will be reviewed.

1.8 Significance of the study

The study will result in faster diagnosis by providing health workers fast access to assistance based on knowledge extracted from various experienced medical workers and knowledge bases.

Fast access to medical help is expected to reduce on delays currently experienced in most hospitals hence improving on overall efficiency of hospital operations.

The government through the ministry of health will be in position of using recommendations from the study on the implementation of CIS in government hospitals.

Training institutions that have always suffered from inadequate staffing, can supplement their man powers with CIS to guide students especially during clerkship

The study will contribute to the available literature on clinical support systems. That can be of help in case of further studies in either the same or related field.

If CISs are finally adopted, medical workers will have their job stress reduced because the system will provide basic support and experts will only be consulted on very complicated issues.

1.9 Operational definitions

A clinical information system; an interactive decision support system designed to assist physicians and other health professionals with decision making tasks.

Software requirement specification; are functions or features that must be included in an information system to satisfy the business need and be acceptable to the users.

System; is an interconnection of various components to perform a specific task.

CHAPTER TWO
LITERATURE REVIEW

This chapter presents a review of literature on topics related to clinical decision support systems. Specific areas covered include; system based clinical support, system requirements, and design techniques and effects of using clinical help systems. Text books, journal articles and newspapers have been synthesized.

According to Leonard and Joseph (2003), decision support systems should provide analysis tools and access to databases in order to support users by providing them with access to decision-oriented information whenever a decision-making situation arises.

2.1 Requirements analysis

According to Ian (2004), requirements discovery includes those techniques used by system analysts to identify or extract system problems and solutions requirements from the user community. According to Sarah and Stacey (2000), there are two categories of system requirements that is to say; functional and non functional requirements. Whitten etal (2001), define functional requirements as features that must be included in an information system to satisfy the business need and be acceptable to the users. Many software developers prefer to preface functional requirements with the word "the system should......X" where X is a deliverable that is measurable. For example; the system should accept user input, the system should print our reports among others.

Likewise, an effective clinical information system should provide medical workers with on-time access to medical knowledge and patients' data to enable them to make more informed decisions. Furthermore, CIS should allow sharing of information. Through the creation of a standard electronic medical record, numerous users involved in the care delivery process can utilize the information stored in the database. This accessibility, allow all users (nurses, administrative staff, laboratory staff, pharmacists, and physicians) to update and extract information for their specific usage needs.

Bryan (2003), on the other hand argues that, non-functional requirements are descriptions of the features or characteristics or attributes of system as well as any constraints that may limit the boundaries of the proposed solution.

According to Kenneth and Jane (2005), DSSs for example CIS, are designed to support unstructured decisions. They are based on the reality that some data must be input to produce information for unstructured decisions. For such systems to do their work, they must poses the following; a knowledge base where expert knowledge is stored and retrieved, a way of capturing or accepting data from its surrounding, and a way of outputting information to the user. These requirements are general to all DSS but specific systems will have different requirements based on the information needs of the users.

Medical diagnosis is a complex human process that is difficult to represent in an algorithmic model. Not only does medical diagnosing require the understanding of symptoms, drug-drug interactions, and patient history, the diagnosing process requires knowledge of diseases in general as well as the general population. CIS utilize varying levels of data in order to diagnose an individual. For example; while one patient may have data showing high cholesterol, chest pain, higher blood pressure within an arterial section, and previous heart attack history within the family, another patient may only show high cholesterol and chest pain. While both patients may require a catheterization, the limited data of the second patient may limit the ability of the diagnosis, and therefore, could lead to the misdiagnosis of the patient.

It is also imperative that the diagnosing systems provide reasoning for the medical diagnosis provided. Such a process would allow the physician to understand the reasons why the system may have made a specific decision.

2.2 System design techniques

According to Bryan (2003), in contrast with requirements analysis, whose concern is what the system should and should not do; design is concerned with how the system will work. Its aim is to transform system requirements into a logical structure that provides an overall picture of how the system works. A range of tools such as entity relation diagrams, data flow diagrams, and data dictionaries, sequence diagrams, and use cases can be used.

There are various system development approaches used in the development of software's. The traditional system development life cycle, prototyping, and computer aided software. According to Whitten etal (2001), The SDLC approach is called cyclical because its phases are executed repeatedly in form of a circle. This approach is suitable for medium sized to large software projects.

Sarah and Stacey (2000), define prototyping as a technique for developing small scale mock-ups which are shown to users to get their feedback. Usually, prototypes are developed at an early stage and they are not intended to be fully functional. The advantage of this method lies in the fact that users don't have to imagine what the system specifications mean in terms of a working and the prototype is changed from time to time until users get satisfied. It is equally important to note that prototyping can only be used for small projects otherwise evaluation of project milestones becomes hard. It is also a costly method because it requires the coming together of analysts, programmers, and software vendor s which is expensive.

CASE tools help in the automation of the often tedious task of documenting entity relationships and data flows in a complex system. Most CASE tools include; project management, data dictionaries, document support, and graphical output. Some even generate prototype code automatically. CASE software is however expensive and requires extensive training to learn and use it.

2.3 The Role of Physicians and Barriers to Use

Anderson J.G (1994) points out that, it is extremely important for physicians, caregivers, staff, administrators, and technical experts to work in collaboration in the design, implementation, and improvement of decision support systems. The physician's role has expanded significantly in today's managed care environment. Physicians and other clinicians need to be involved throughout the whole process of finding, designing, implementing, and improving such a system. Their input and support is critical because of the significant role that physicians play in the health care delivery process. The acceptance of these systems has not been easy. One reason for this is the fact that these systems affect the long history of traditional medical practices.

According to Institute of Medicine, Division of Health Care Services (1997), failure to accept these systems among physicians occurs when implementation does not provide direct benefits to their work and especially when the process of implementing CIS changes the traditional practices of the clinical environment.

2.4 Benefits of the Clinical Information Systems

According to Tang and McDonald (2001), the primary benefit of the clinical information system will be within the domains of task support and decision support. The task support field has been revolutionalized through the implementation an electronic medical record. The universalization of the electronic medical record will increases the accessibility of patient information by clinicians as well as increases the amount of data available for clinical use, reducing medical error significantly.

In addition, the development of the clinical information system arose due to a need to maintain clinical management control. This management of clinical practice is applicable to individual patient management, intra-practice management, and inter-practice management. On an individual patient basis, the measurement of quality of care, the monitoring of care provided, and feedback regarding the care that has been provided allows for improved quality care provision. A CIS would allow for the maintenance of a standard practice pattern, which includes the provision of care based on specified care paths and/or flow sheets. Furthermore, the treatments and protocols chosen for care provision can be compared to an industry standard, or a "best practice" methodology.

Clinical decision support software offers the possibility to improve the quality and reduce the cost of care by influencing medical decisions at the time and place that these decisions are made. An ideal CIS would alert physicians when outlier results are returned from data entry of laboratory testing. The data attained for a specific patient can then be compared to the general population to indicate whether the data is within the normal fit or is an outlier that may require further analysis. Such a practice would induce the physician to notice certain data that may otherwise go unnoticed, and therefore, alter the diagnosis of the patient.

Furthermore, physician especially trainees (interns) may interact with the system on a hypothesis-testing basis. A physician may enter a possible diagnosis into the system and then receive feedback from the system regarding the plausibility of such a diagnosis being true. This allows physicians to receive guided feedback during their consideration of similar diagnoses, which may be significantly different based on their appropriate care path.

In a study carried out by Thomas, Ramnarayan, Michael, Prabhat, Wilson, Emily , (...) and Joseph B (2008), it was demonstrated that, approximately 20% of critically ill children will be admitted without an established diagnosis and that the clinical team makes an accurate Preliminary diagnosis almost 90% of the time. This rate is improved by use of the ISABEL tool as well as a higher degree of clinical training and experience. While this might be true in some instances, such as the prevention of medication errors, there is evidence that increased need for technology may also lead to increased patient harm. For example, too much of x-rays is lethal. They attributed Isabel's success to its uniqueness. ISABEL is a unique System that collects data from multiple sources including textbooks, journal articles and reviews to generate a potential diagnostic list for the user. ISABEL has been shown to be an effective reminding system in adult emergency departments, with 95% accuracy in presenting the user with the final diagnosis and 90% accuracy in obtaining "must-not-miss" diagnoses. The most interesting question is whether clinicians can improve their own diagnostic ability in collaboration with the use of ISABEL? The answer lies with Kenneth & Jane (2005) who argue that, DSSs aid decision making by providing access to information in a more customized manner and this makes it easy for clinicians to learn and to use.

According to Taylor (2006), many patients mistakenly believe that their physicians are omniscient just as many physicians think that their patients are ignorant. Recognition of these mistakes has led, in recent years, to the development of the idea of shared decision making which is made possible through the use of CIS. A 2005 systematic review by Garg et al. of 100 studies concluded that CDSs improved practitioner performance in 64% of the studies. The CDSs improved patient outcomes in 13% of the studies. Sustainable CDSs features associated with improved practitioner performance include automatic electronic prompts rather than requiring user activation of the system. Garg et al. concluded that the number and methodological quality of studies have improved from 1973 through 2004. Another 2005 systematic review of 70 studies by Kawamoto et al. found that; "Decision support systems significantly improved clinical practice in 68% of trials." For example, Physicians at the university of North Carolina (UNC) medical center, one of the world's leading telemedicine centers, use computer network connections and sophisticated imaging technologies to extend specialist's expertise into rural and remote areas, where such expertise isn't readily available. In one recent case, a young child living in an isolated rural community suffered a brain hemorrhage and couldn't be moved. A local surgeon uploaded x-rays of the girl's brain and consulted with UNC neurologist. The surgery was a success.

According to Floyd (2002), CDSSs could bring dramatic quality gains to health care systems by making specialized expertise available at low cost. For example, according to Bryan (2003), technology's possibilities were demonstrated during President Clinton's visit in 1998 to china. Stanford University consulted with Chinese doctors on a treatment plan for two seriously I'll children located in a remote region of western china and the operation was successful. Despite this great sounding, some major problems will have to be solved before its use becomes widespread. For example, state licensing programs forbid doctors to practice medicine outside the state in which they were licensed and if a patient is misdiagnosed and then claims that face-to-face meeting would have prevented the misdiagnosis, a malpractice lawsuit could result

Clinical management support also applies to inter-practice management situations. By standardizing "best practice" care methodologies; the clinician has a database against which their care path decision may be measured. Also, the integration of the numerous care contributors into a single information system will allow for cost management and quality control across hospitals.

CIS bring about competition support; the development of an effective clinical information system places health care organizations in an advantageous position relative to other competitors. The benefits of a clinical information system are evident in terms of the reduction of medical error, the standardization of medical protocol, knowledge sharing, cost control, quality control, and decision support. Therefore, firms that are able to develop facilities in these areas will have a competitive edge over other care delivery organizations.

Clinical information system I allow for the comparison of numerical data from numerous fields with the data obtained from other firms in the industry. Such comparisons allow delivery organizations to increase the quality of care accordingly, learn from other firms, adjust price according to competitor levels, and adjust to community demand levels.

CHAPTER THREE
METHODOLOGY

This chapter presents tools, techniques, and methodologies that were used to develop a computer based clinical help system. It covers the research design, the study population, sample size, research instruments, and procedure for data collection among others.

3.1 Research Design

A cross-sectional survey and interviews will be used in this study. It has been selected due to its appropriateness in situations where the population is very large and generalization is required. The theme of the study is whether clinical information systems can provide adequate support to perform clinical tasks. This will be done through evaluation of the effects of clinical information systems on the quality of healthcare. The need to adopt CISs is to respond to the perceived wanting situation in hospitals that lack adequate human resource to attend to patients and to give adequate guidance to medical trainees to learn and treat patients effectively. The population of study will include people with formal medical knowledge, specifically; doctors, nurses, and interns and hospital management staff working with regional referral hospitals. In Uganda, there are twelve regional referral hospitals found in the following districts; Arua, fort portal, Gulu, Hoima ,Jinja ,Kabale, Lira ,Masaka ,Mbale ,Soroti and Mubende . This population is appropriate because; it covers the whole of Uganda and therefore the outcomes can be generalized to represent the whole of Uganda, all regional hospitals in Uganda have all the five target categories of people that is to say doctors, clinicians, nurses, trainees, and administrative staff. , there is little beuaracracy in government hospitals compared to private hospitals, and lastly it is in government hospitals that complaints of low pay and understaffing are most pronounced. Purposive sampling will be used select respondents. Data will be collected using questionnaires and interviews. Analysis of this data will be done using spss and the rank correlation coefficient, khi square will be calculated to see the extent to which the outcomes from the two data collection methods and the relationship between health workers' attitude and success of CIS.

3.2 Study population

The study population is composed of; medical doctors, allied health clinicians, nurses, dentists and medical trainees, working in government regional referral hospitals.

Figure 3.1: showing the distribution of hospitals in Uganda

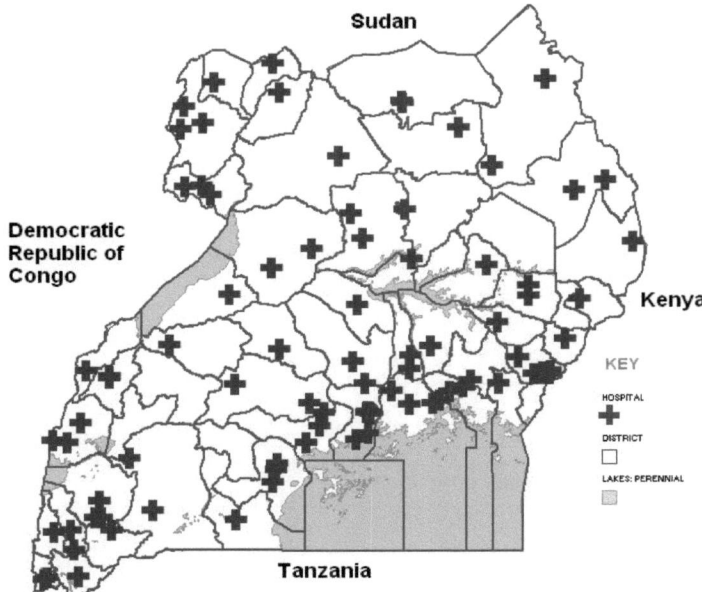

The hospitals indicated above include both district and regional referral hospitals.

Table 3.1: The table below shows Health workers at national level

Medical doctors	3361
Nurses and midwifery professionals	664
Dentists	98
Pharmacists	162
Other health professionals	3572
Allied health clinical	4378
Nurses and midwifery associate professionals	20340
Allied health dental	342
Allied health pharmacy	600
Allied health diagnostic	1622
Other allied health associate professionals	5 828
Nurse assistant/aid	16 621
Traditional medicine practitioners and faith healers	5 430
Accounts and finance professionals	159
Accounts and finance associate professionals	278
Clerks	437
Technical and engineering professionals	12
Engineering technicians	129
Non-health professional	452
Other non-health associate professional	664
Support staff	962
TOTAL 66 111	**66111**

Source: MoH, analysis of census data, 2005.

Compared to other sub-Saharan African countries the ratios in the above table compare relatively well. The above table however, reveals that support staff clinical workers (including nursing aids / Assistants) working in the health sector form approximately one third of the whole workforce (excluding traditional and faith healers). These health workers are not appropriately trained yet a large proportion of the population exclusively depends on them particularly in the rural areas of the country. In this study, our emphasis is on doctors, nurses, and clinicians because these are people who in most hospitals and especially at regional hospitals involved in the diagnosis of patients. Thus taking 3361 for doctors, 4378 for clinicians and 664 for nurses. In total we get 8403. The total of 8403 is as per the year 2005. Let us round it off to 9000 to cater for the new medical personnel that might have been added and some other health workers like dentists, associate nurses and interns. Hence our population of study is estimated to be 9000.

Let us make another assumption that these health workers are equally distributed amongst the 12 regional hospitals.

Table 3.2: Table showing the estimated total population stratified

Title	frequency
Doctors	3361
clinicians	4378
nurses	664
others	597
Total	**9000**

3.3 Target Sample

383 people will be considered in the study. Yamane (1967:886) provides a simplified formula to calculate sample sizes. This formula was used to calculate the sample size. From every hospital selected, 31 respondents will be selected.

Equation 3: $$n = \frac{N}{1 + N(e)^2}$$

Figure 3.2: showing Yamane's formula for calculating target

a 95% confidence level and P =0.5 will be used.

3.3.1 Sampling procedure

Research assistants or the researcher himself will go to the respective regional referral hospitals as listed in the research design. At every hospital, the researcher will select medical workers with various professions (doctors/dentists, nurses (nursing officers preferable), clinicians). Those with a bachelor's degree in (medicine, allied health clinical, nursing, and dentistry) will be given first priority. A starting (initial) hospital will randomly be selected from the list and then a heuristic function called the" nearest neighbor" will be used to select the next hospital. This will be repeated until all government regional referral hospitals are completed.

3.4 Data collection tools

Questionnaire and interview will be used to gather data. Fixed format, multiple choices formats and one or two open ended questions will make the instrument easy to complete and ensure that respondents remain within the boundaries of the study scope and ease data analysis. While designing the questionnaire, anonymity of respondents was upheld in order to elicit more satisfactory information. This claim is corroborated by the assertion of Amin (1990:198) when he stated that questionnaires are preferable since they avoid the embarrassment of direct questioning and so enhance the validity of responses. It was intended that, the questionnaires would be easy to understand and complete. The questionnaire items were developed based on the objectives of the study. Since the population and corresponding sample size is large and sparsely distributed all over Uganda, the questionnaire technique will be the main data collection tool. However, interviews will also be conducted alongside questionnaires to validate data collected using questionnaires.

3.5 Scoring of the scale

When using the likert-scale, scoring must be consistent. Thus if it is decided that on a positive statement a high score of 5 is for Strongly Agree, then a score of 1 should be for Strongly Disagree or Negative statements must be scored with a 1 for Strongly Agree and a 5 for Strongly Disagree. Such reversals are important to take note of. On the Likert-type scale constructed for this particular study, responses will be graded for each statement, and will be expressed in terms of the following five categories, SA; A; U; D and SD. (SA) for Strongly Agree, (A) for Agree, (U) for undecided, (D) for Disagree and (SD) for Strongly Disagree. The statements will either be positive or negative. To score the scale, the responses will be credited 5; 4; 3; 2 and 1 respectively. The sum of the item credits represented the individual's total score. Scoring keys were made in order to ease the scoring procedure.

3.6 Validity and reliability of the instrument

In an article by Lozano, Garcia-Cueto and Muniz (2008), two psychometric properties, i.e. reliability and validity will depend on the best number of options for the Likert scale. Between 4 and 7 is appropriate while More than 7 options will give better psychometric properties, but one has to make sure that it will not exceed the discriminative capacity of the respondents. A reliability coefficient of .85 is often achieved. By using the internal-consistency method of item selection, the scale approaches uni-dimensionality in many cases. As a whole however, a lot of thought has been given to the design of the instrument that is by ensuring that every item in the questionnaire measures an aspect related to an objective of the study and up to five options have been provided for 90% of the items in the questionnaire. A focused group of five master's holders and assistant lecturer at the KIU checked the content validity of the instrument. To further enhance the reliability of this instrument, triangulation will be used. Health workers willing to help in further research will be interviewed two weeks after the return of questionnaires. The number to be interviewed will be a sample of the total number of such respondents and this number will be calculated using Yamane's formula. Similar questions as those asked in the questionnaire will for a schedule. A statistical spearman's rank correlation coefficient ($r=1-(6\Sigma d^2)/n\ (n^2-1)$) will be calculated for questions that seek direct answers to research questions. The value got will be a representation of the extent to which the instrument is reliable. Purposive sampling and face validity will be used in selection and determination of whom to interview.

3.7 Data Gathering Procedures

Prior to the study, an introductory letter will be got from the school of post graduate studies and research. The purpose of this letter will be to introduce the researcher to the management of selected hospitals. After arriving at the hospital, the researcher will introduce himself to the hospital administrator and request for permission to collect data at the hospital a date convenient for the hospital staff will be set. The researcher will distribute questionnaires to 31 respondents per hospital. After the questionnaires have been returned, the researcher will check for those respondents (doctor, clinicians and nurses) that have offered to volunteer in further research. He will contact them by e-mail and arrange for an interview. On the agreed date, the researcher will move to the respondent's premises and hold an interview session with respondents. Similar questions to those administered in the questionnaire will be allowed. However, respondents will be allowed to provide additional data in case they wish to.

3.8 Data Analysis

Descriptive statistics will be used to analyze data. Minor gaps in the questionnaires will be dealt with in a focused group discussions this will involve resolving hand writing issues, dealing with unfilled gaps among others. Data will be entered into the spss and Frequencies, means, spearman's rank correlations will be generated and variances will be calculated.

3.8 Ethical Considerations

According to Charema (2004), Informed consent will be sought before the actual collection of data. The research will thoroughly explain to the respondents the purpose of the study and request for their voluntary participation in the study. ethics is the philosophical study of moral value of human conduct and of the rules and principles that ought to govern it, or a code of behavior considered correct especially that of a particular group, profession or individual. It also involves the moral fitness of a decision and course of action taken (Capuzzi and Gross, 2006). The 1974 Federal Privacy Act restricts access to medical information and records. Therefore, clinicians have a duty to protect identifiable individuals from any serious threat of harm if they have information that could prevent the harm. As mentioned above, the determining factor in justifying breaking confidentiality is whether there is good reason to believe specific individuals (or groups) are placed in serious danger depending on the medical information needed. The most famous case of this sort of exception is that of homicidal ideation, when the patient shares a specific plan with a physician or psychotherapist to harm a particular individual. The court has required that traditional patient confidentiality be breached in these sorts of cases. Research implies making results public.

According to American Counseling Association (1996), Autonomy is the principle that addresses the concept of independence. The essence of this principle is allowing an individual the freedom of choice and action. It addresses the responsibility of the counselor to encourage clients, when appropriate, to make their own decisions and to act on their own values. Since medical information should be kept secret and research a public affair, ethics become the guiding principle that ensures the protection of the respondent as a participant in the research process. However, it is in the interest of every research to make his/her finding published. Thus it is ethical for every researcher to discuss his/her study limitations and problems experienced during data collection and how these problems impacted on the quality of conclusions drawn from the results.

Anonymity and confidentiality of individual contributions will be upheld such that; All respondents will be informed of confidentiality of the information they provide and their anonymity to the public. To ensure that, respondents shall not provide names, personal phone numbers and any other identification. Questionnaires will be given serial numbers which might be used for reference in case the researcher intends to make a follow-up. The hospital's info email address will be used together with questionnaire serial numbers.

3.9 Limitations of the study

The population is sparsely scattered all over Uganda and thus moving to all those places is likely to a problem due to time and transport costs and or unavailability. Where the researcher cannot physically reach due some circumstances, the questionnaires will be posted and additional follow-up will be done on phone.

Most medicals professional especially in Africa still don't accept that IT in medicine can enhance their performance thus they may respond in such away to despise the applicability of CIS (Taylor, 2006).

References

American Counseling Association (2005). Code of Ethics. Alexandria, VA: Author.

Anderson JG. Computer-based patient records and changing physician practice patterns. Top in Health Information Manage 1994; 15: 10-23.

Androulidakis, A., Nielsen, A.D., Adriana, P. & Dimitris, K. (2006) Technology and health care. *Journal of the European Society for Engineering and Medicine* 14(3).

Association of American Medical Colleges. Calls for restoration of BBA Medicare cuts to teaching Hospitals.

Babour, R. S. (1998). Mixing qualitative methods: Quality assurance or qualitative quagmire? *Qualitative Health Research, 8*(3), 352-361.

Bryan P. (2003). *Computers in your future 2003; Committed to shaping the next generation of IT experts.* (5th Ed). New York: Prentice Hall.

Capuzzi, D. & Gross, D. R. (2006) Introduction to Group Counseling .Denver, CO: Love Publishing.

Charema, J (2004), the present system of guidance and counseling by individuals and/organizations in Zimbabwe. University of Pretoria etd.

Cohen, L. & Holliday, M. (1982). *Statistics for Social Scientists.* London: Harper and Row.

Floyd, F. (2002). *Computers: Navigating change.* EMC/Paradigm publishing.

Gluud, C. & Nikolova, D. (2007). *Likely country of origin in publications on randomized controlled trials and controlled clinical trials during the last 60 years.* Doi: id=17326823

Ian, S. (2004). *Software Engineering.* (7th Ed). New York, NY: Addison-Wesley.

Institute of Medicine, Division of Health Care Services, Committee on Improving the Patient Record (1997). The computer-based patient record: *an essential technology for health care*. Revised edition. Washington (DC): National Academy Press;

Joseph, R., Cissy, L., Mbasaalaki-Mwaka & Grace, N. (2010). Challenges faced by health workers in providing counseling services to HIV-positive children in Uganda. *Journal of the International AIDS Society.*

Kawamoto, K., Caitlin, A., Houlihan, E., Andrew, B., David, F. & Lobach (2005). Improving clinical practice using clinical decision support systems: *a systematic review of trials to identify features critical to success.*

Kenneth C. & Jane, P. (2005). *Management Information Systems: Managing the Digital Firm* (9th Ed.). New York, NY: Prentice Hall; Pearson Education.

Leonard, J. & Joseph, V. (2003). *Information Systems Today.* Prentice hall, Inc.

Lozano, L.M., Garcia-Cueto, E., and Muniz, J. (2008). Effect of the number of response categories on the reliability and validity of rating scales.

Sarah, E.H. & Stacey, C.S. (2000) *Computers, Communications, and Information: A user's introduction; Comprehensive version* (7th Ed). New York: McGraw-Hill.

Tang PC, McDonald CJ. (2001) *Computer-based patient-record systems.* In: Shortliffe EH, Perreault LE, editors. Medical informatics: computer applications in health care and biomedicine. 2nd Ed. New York: Springer-Verlag; p 327-58

Taylor, P. (2006*). From patient data to medical knowledge: The principles and practice of health informatics*. London, England: Blackwell.

Thomas, N.J., Ramnarayan, P., Michael J. B., Prabhat M., Wilson, S., Emily B. N., (...) & Joseph B. (2008). An international assessment of a web-based diagnostic tool in critically ill children. *Technology and Health Care* (16) 103.

Whitten, J.L., Bentley, L.D. & Dittman. K.C. (2001). *Systems analysis and design methods* (7th Ed.). New York: McGraw-Hill: IRWIN.

Wilber, M. (2010). The weekly observer. *KIU opens teaching hospital in Kenya*. November, 28 2010.

APPENDIX II
QUESTIONAIRE

Preamble:

Dear respondent, am by the names of Alikira Richard a PhD student of Management of information systems at Kampala international university. It is a requirement that every student carries out a study aimed at solving a specific problem. My study title is **adoption of clinical information system in Uganda**. You have bee purposively chosen to support me in this study by answering questions that follow. All responses will be handled with utmost faith and confidentiality.

Ethical consideration

I understand the purpose and significance of this study. I have not been coerced to take part in this study. And I have been assured of privacy of the information provided

----

Signature

(Tick in the checkbox that best describes you)

Part 1: personal details

Write your initials

....

Gender:

Male ☐ Female ☐

What is your Profession?

Doctor ☐ nurse ☐ clinician ☐ intern ☐ other ☐

How many years of experience do you have?

0-1 ☐
2-4 ☐
5-10 ☐
Above 10 ☐

What is you highest Academic qualification?

Certificate ☐ Diploma ☐ Bachelor ☐ Masters ☐ PhD ☐

Part 2: About the system

SA = strongly agree (you strongly support the idea)

AG = agree (you do support but little doubt)

U= undecided (not sure)

D= disagree (do not support the idea)

SD= strongly agree (you strongly don't support)

"A clinical information system is a collection of various information technology applications that provides a centralized repository of information related to patient care across distributed locations"

(Tick in the box that best describes your attitude)

Section A. Software requirements specification

The system should	SA	A	U	D	SD
1. Capture patient's data					
2. Allow users to login with password					
3. Provide just in time help					
4. Provide access to patient data					
5. Provide access to expert knowledge					
6. Generate patient data reports					
7. Prescribe drugs for patients					
8. suggest diagnosis					
9. Guide operation in theatre					
10. should alert users using audio beeps					
11. store patient's data					
12. Guide patients on treatment					

Section B: Effects of clinical information systems (CIS)

The following are effects of clinical information systems;	SA	A	U	D	SD
1. will replace health workers in the near future					
2. are used by patients to get correct treatment					
3. Medical workers can consult CIS the same way they do to consultants					
4. Give case specific advise					
5. Can reduce on the cost of operation					
6. Make Health workers more productive					
7. Increases the speed of students in carrying out diagnosis					

P.T.O.

Section C: Roles of medical worker in CIS

Health workers ;	SA	A	U	D	SD
1. provide knowledge used by these systems					
2. use the system during diagnosis					
3. Respond to warnings from the system					
4. Input patient data					
5. Verify reports generated by the system					
6. Guide diagnosis					
7. Prescribe drugs based on results from the system					

Section D: System design techniques (tick where appropriate)

The design of the system should;	SA	A	U	D	SD
1. Use a Graphical user interface					
2. Use the traditional system development life cycle					
3. Use Prototyping					
4. System design should make use of use case diagrams					
5. Use data flow diagrams to how data moves through the system					

SECTION E: contingency questions

1. Does the hospital you work for have any form of CIS   [ ] Yes   [ ] No
2. Have you ever used a clinical information system?   [ ] Yes   [ ] No
3. Based on the above, should clinical information systems be adopted?   [ ] Yes   [ ] No

Write any additional information that you think might be of help to the study……………………………………………………………………………………………………
………………………………………………………………………………………………………

Thank you